A Complete Guide To Understanding and Managing Coronary Artery Disease (CAD)

Empowering Strategies for a Heart Healthy Lifestyle, from Prevention to Emotional Well-being

Maggie E. McDonald

Table Of Contents

Introduction

Coronary Artery Disease (CAD) is a frequent and potentially dangerous cardiac ailment defined by the inadequate delivery of blood, oxygen, and nutrients to the heart muscle due to the narrowing of the coronary arteries. These critical blood channels are important for guaranteeing the heart's normal function, and when cholesterol deposits and inflammation obstruct them, the outcome is coronary artery disease.

At its heart, CAD includes the deposition of lipids, cholesterol, and other substances on the inner walls of the coronary arteries, a process known as atherosclerosis. This deposit, referred to as plaque, not only narrows the arteries, reducing blood flow but can also burst, leading to the production of blood clots. This dual process offers a serious hazard to heart health, with the potential to induce chest discomfort (angina), shortness of breath, and, in severe situations, a heart attack.

Atherosclerosis, the fundamental process of CAD, is the condition in which the inner walls of the heart arteries get covered with a film of plaque. This accumulation triggers a cascade of actions, ultimately reducing blood flow to the heart. Plaque can not only constrict arteries but can also burst, prompting the production of blood clots. This approach is crucial to knowing the mechanics that drive CAD.

Importance of Managing CAD for a Healthy Life

The necessity of effectively managing CAD cannot be emphasized. This problem, frequently accumulating over decades, may go undiscovered until a substantial blockage occurs, resulting in severe symptoms or a heart attack. Therefore, knowing and managing the risk factors and symptoms are vital for preventing problems and maintaining a healthy life.

Signs and Symptoms:

The indications and symptoms of CAD are various and might include chest discomfort or angina, shortness of breath, and exhaustion. Recognizing these indications is crucial for obtaining timely medical help. In certain situations, CAD can emerge as a heart attack, with traditional indications such as crushing chest pain, shoulder or arm discomfort, shortness of breath, and perspiration. Notably, women may report uncommon symptoms, such as neck or jaw discomfort, nausea, and exhaustion.

When to Seek Medical Help:

Immediate intervention is needed if there's a suspicion of a heart attack. Calling medical assistance. Risk factors such as smoking, high blood pressure, high cholesterol, diabetes, obesity, and a family history of heart disease increase the probability of CAD. If one falls into these high-risk groups, getting medical guidance and appropriate testing for early identification is crucial.

Understanding CAD's complexity is the first step toward good management. Recognizing the indications, eliminating risk factors, and obtaining prompt medical treatment is crucial in navigating this cardiovascular issue. The following parts will go deeper into the causes, risk factors, symptoms, diagnosis, and techniques to successfully treat and prevent CAD for a better and more meaningful life.

Understanding Coronary Artery Disease (CAD)

Coronary Artery Disease (CAD) is a complicated cardiovascular illness that includes the insufficient flow of blood to the heart muscle, resulting in a range of symptoms and severe problems. To appreciate CAD thoroughly, it's necessary to investigate its description, causes, the development of atherosclerosis, and the many risk factors linked with this ailment.

Definition and Explanation of CAD

Coronary Artery Disease, also referred to as coronary heart disease, is a medical disorder where the coronary arteries, responsible for transporting oxygen-rich blood to the heart muscle, become restricted or clogged. This constriction is often caused by the deposition of cholesterol deposits and plaques on the inner walls of these arteries. The effect is decreased blood flow, which can result in chest discomfort (angina), shortness of breath, and in severe circumstances, lead to a heart attack.

Understanding CAD entails identifying it as a gradual disorder that develops over time, sometimes without visible symptoms until a severe blockage occurs. The recognition of this trend is crucial for early intervention and successful management.

Causes of CAD

1. Cholesterol Deposits and Plaques:

One of the key causes of CAD is the slow development of cholesterol deposits and plaques within the coronary arteries. Cholesterol, a fatty substance, can build on the arterial walls, producing plaques over time. As these plaques form, they restrict the arteries, limiting the smooth flow of blood. If a plaque ruptures, it might induce the production of blood clots, leading to additional obstructions and problems.

2. Inflammation in the Heart Arteries:

Inflammation has a crucial impact in the development and progression of CAD. Chronic inflammation can damage the inner lining of the coronary arteries, making them more vulnerable to the buildup of cholesterol and the creation of plaques. Inflammatory activities contribute to the fragility of these plaques, increasing the risk of rupture and blood clot development.

Development of Atherosclerosis

1. Explanation of Atherosclerosis:

Atherosclerosis is the underlying mechanism in CAD and entails the progressive thickening and hardness of the artery walls owing to the development of plaques. This disorder impairs the flexibility and function of the arteries, resulting in diminished blood flow. Atherosclerosis is a systemic disease that may damage arteries throughout the body, but its influence on the coronary arteries is particularly essential owing to its function in giving oxygen to the heart.

2. Formation and Impact of Plaque:

Plaque formation is a dynamic process. It starts with the deposition of cholesterol, lipids, and cellular debris on the arterial walls. Over time, this deposit matures into plaques, which may be firm and solid or fragile and sensitive to rupture. The impact of plaque goes beyond narrowing the arteries; it can lead to the production of blood clots, abrupt blockages, and reduced blood flow to the heart muscle.

Risk Factors

1. Common Risk Factors (Smoking, High Blood Pressure, Diabetes):

- Smoking: Tobacco smoke includes toxic substances that can damage blood vessels and accelerate the deposition of plaque.
- High Blood Pressure: Elevated blood pressure exerts stress on the artery walls, adding to their hardening and constriction.
- Diabetes: Diabetes is related to metabolic alterations that raise the risk of atherosclerosis and CAD.

2. Less Common Risk Factors (Sleep Apnea, High Sensitivity C Reactive Protein):

- Sleep Apnea: Interruptions in breathing during sleep, characteristic of sleep apnea, might contribute to hypertension and raise CAD risk.
- High Sensitivity C Reactive Protein (hs CRP): Elevated levels of this protein suggest inflammation and can serve as a marker for increased cardiovascular risk.

Understanding these causes and risk factors is crucial to both prevention and therapy. In the coming parts, we will look into the signs and symptoms of CAD, diagnosis, and effective measures for living with and avoiding this cardiovascular ailment.

Signs and Symptoms of (CAD)

Understanding the signs and symptoms of Coronary Artery Disease (CAD) is crucial for early identification and appropriate therapy. CAD commonly appears through different signs, ranging from traditional chest discomfort (angina) to more subtle symptoms, such as exhaustion and shortness of breath. Recognizing these indicators is vital for obtaining appropriate medical assistance and implementing required lifestyle modifications.

Chest Pain (Angina)

1. Description and Types of Chest Pain:

Chest discomfort, or angina, is a defining sign of CAD. The pain might appear in numerous ways, and knowing these variances is critical for correct diagnosis.

Stable Angina: This is the most prevalent kind of angina. It happens after physical exertion or situations of stress and is often predictable. The discomfort is commonly characterized as a pressure or squeezing sensation in the chest.

Unstable Angina: Unlike stable angina, unstable angina is unexpected and can develop at rest. The pain may be more acute and protracted, signifying an increased risk of a heart attack.

Variant Angina (Prinzmetal's Angina): This variety is produced by a spasm in the coronary arteries, resulting in transient blood flow restriction. It commonly happens at rest and can be severe.

2. Triggers and Duration:

Angina can be induced by different situations, and knowing these triggers assists in controlling the problem.

Physical Activity: Exertion or tension during activities might trigger angina.

Emotional Stress: Intense emotions might be a cause for angina events.

Exposure to Cold: Cold temperatures or other conditions producing vasoconstriction may trigger angina.

The length of angina bouts varies. They normally linger for a few minutes and diminish with rest or treatment. Prolonged or intense pain may suggest a more grave situation.

Shortness of Breath

Shortness of breath, medically termed dyspnea, is another typical symptom of CAD. Reduced blood supply to the heart affects its capacity to pump properly, resulting in a sense of breathlessness. This symptom can occur during physical activity or even during rest, depending on the severity of CAD.

Understanding the association between shortness of breath and CAD is crucial. Individuals suffering inexplicable and persistent breathlessness should seek medical assistance soon. It might be an indication of poor cardiac function that requires examination and intervention.

Fatigue

Fatigue, or unusual fatigue, is a modest yet significant symptom of CAD. When the heart fails to pump adequate blood to fulfill the body's demands, individuals may suffer chronic weariness. This weariness is not usually eased by rest and might impair everyday activities and quality of life.

Recognizing the relationship between tiredness and CAD is critical for early management. Addressing the underlying cardiovascular disorders through lifestyle modifications and medical care can frequently ease tiredness and enhance general well-being.

Heart Attack

1. Classic Signs and Symptoms:

A heart attack, or myocardial infarction, happens when there is a total blockage of blood flow to a segment of the heart muscle. Recognizing the traditional signs and symptoms is crucial for obtaining quick medical treatment.

- Crushing Chest Pain or Pressure: The pain may extend to the arms, jaw, or back.
- Shortness of Breath: Difficulty breathing is a typical concomitant symptom.
- Sweating: Profuse sweating sometimes follows a heart attack.

2. Atypical Symptoms, Especially in Women:
While men and women share many common heart attack symptoms, women may have unique signs.

- Neck, Jaw, or Back discomfort: Women may feel discomfort in regions other than the chest.
- Nausea or Vomiting: Digestive problems might be more prevalent in women.
- Weariness: Unexplained weariness may be a warning indication for women.

Recognizing these unusual symptoms is critical, as women may not always present with traditional chest discomfort. Understanding the variability in how heart attacks appear in various individuals is vital for early medical intervention.

In conclusion, being aware of the signs and symptoms linked with CAD is the first step toward proactive heart health. Whether it's chest discomfort, shortness of breath, exhaustion, or the more important signs of a heart attack, early detection, and immediate action are vital for successful management and improved results. In the coming parts, we will investigate the diagnostic processes for CAD and dig into living with and avoiding this cardiovascular ailment.

Diagnosis and When to Seek Medical Help

Coronary Artery Disease (CAD) is a complicated cardiovascular disorder that requires early identification for optimal care. Understanding the importance of early diagnosis and the diagnostic tests available is vital for persons at risk or experiencing symptoms suggestive of CAD.

Importance of Early Detection

The value of early identification in CAD cannot be emphasized. Detecting and diagnosing CAD in its early stages can lead to improved results and the deployment of prompt therapies. Early identification allows for the commencement of appropriate medical therapies, lifestyle adjustments, and preventative measures to limit the course of the condition and lower the risk of consequences such as heart attacks.

CAD frequently develops over a lengthy time, and symptoms may not show until the problem has progressed. Therefore, frequent health checkups and knowledge of risk factors are crucial. If individuals develop symptoms such as chest discomfort, shortness of breath, or exhaustion, obtaining early medical assistance is vital. Early identification not only increases the efficacy of therapy but also promotes the overall quality of life by treating the fundamental causes of the condition.

Diagnostic Tests for CAD

1. Angiography:

Angiography is a crucial diagnostic method for assessing the status of the coronary arteries. This imaging technology offers precise pictures of the blood vessels, allowing healthcare practitioners to discover blockages, narrowings, or other abnormalities in the coronary arteries.

During coronary angiography, a contrast dye is injected into the arteries, and X-ray imaging catches the flow of blood. This gives a full look at the coronary arteries' anatomy and any potential blockages.

Angiography is commonly used when CAD is suspected or to examine the degree of existing coronary artery blockages. The results aid healthcare practitioners in identifying the most suitable course of therapy, whether it be medicinal management, angioplasty, or coronary artery bypass surgery.

2. Blood Tests:

Blood tests play a significant part in detecting CAD by examining several indicators that suggest cardiac health and possible concerns. Common blood tests include:

Lipid Profile: Measures levels of cholesterol, including low-density lipoprotein (LDL) and high-density lipoprotein (HDL), offering insights into the risk of atherosclerosis and CAD.

Troponin Test: Detects troponin, a protein released into the circulation when there is damage to the heart muscle, assisting in the diagnosis of a heart attack.

C reactive Protein (CRP) Test: Measures inflammation, which is related to the development and progression of CAD.

These blood tests contribute to a thorough assessment of heart health, enabling healthcare practitioners to understand the risk factors and potential consequences associated with CAD.

3. Stress Tests:

Stress tests are diagnostic procedures that measure how the heart operates under increasing strain and stress. These tests are important in diagnosing CAD related abnormalities that may not be obvious under resting situations. Common types of stress testing include:

Exertion Stress Test: Involves physical exertion on a treadmill or stationary bicycle while measuring heart rate, blood pressure, and electrocardiogram (ECG) changes.

Nuclear Stress Test: Combines a stress test with the injection of a small quantity of radioactive material to generate pictures of blood flow to the heart.

Stress Echocardiography: Utilizes ultrasound imaging to monitor heart function and blood flow before and after stress.

Stress tests let healthcare doctors analyze the heart's reaction to physical activity, detect regions with restricted blood flow, and establish the overall cardiovascular health of the patient.

These diagnostic tests, when utilized in combination, offer a full picture of the patient's cardiovascular health. Early diagnosis using these tests helps healthcare practitioners to adapt therapies, whether through drugs, lifestyle adjustments, or invasive procedures, to match the particular requirements of patients with CAD.

Recognizing the need for early detection and performing suitable diagnostic procedures are crucial stages in controlling Coronary Artery Disease.

Seeking medical treatment when symptoms emerge or when at risk owing to variables such as age, family history, or lifestyle choices is critical for prompt management and improved results. The next parts will dig into living with CAD, including lifestyle adjustments, medicines, and preventative techniques for a heart-healthy life.

Living with Coronary Artery Disease (CAD)

Living with Coronary Artery Disease (CAD) involves a comprehensive approach that incorporates lifestyle adjustments, medication management, and a dedication to heart-healthy habits. Individuals diagnosed with CAD can dramatically enhance their quality of life and lower the risk of problems by embracing good behaviors and following prescribed medical treatments.

Lifestyle Changes

1. Quitting Smoking:

Smoking is a major risk factor for CAD, as the chemicals in tobacco smoke can damage blood vessels and hasten the onset of atherosclerosis. Quitting smoking is one of the most important lifestyle improvements for patients with CAD.

The advantages of smoking cessation are extensive and extend beyond cardiovascular health. Within just a few weeks of quitting, blood pressure falls, circulation improves, and the risk of heart attack begins to reduce. Support from healthcare specialists, smoking cessation programs, and behavioral therapies can benefit individuals in overcoming nicotine addiction.

2. Managing High Blood Pressure, Cholesterol, and Diabetes:

Effectively treating hypertension, high cholesterol, and diabetes is crucial to CAD treatment. High blood pressure and increased cholesterol levels contribute to the advancement of atherosclerosis, whereas diabetes is a substantial risk factor for cardiovascular disease.

Medications, as given by healthcare practitioners, play a key role in regulating these disorders. Additionally, lifestyle improvements such as a heart-healthy diet, frequent exercise, and stress management are critical components in managing blood pressure, cholesterol, and diabetes. Regular monitoring and contact with healthcare specialists are crucial for changing treatment strategies depending on individual reactions.

3. Regular Exercise:

Physical exercise is a cornerstone of living well with CAD. Regular exercise helps strengthen the heart, improve circulation, and contribute to overall cardiovascular health. Engaging in activities like walking, swimming, or cycling for at least 150 minutes each week is suggested.

Exercise plans should be adjusted to individual fitness levels and interests. Healthcare practitioners can facilitate the establishment of a safe and successful fitness regimen. Regular physical exercise not only improves the heart but also aids weight control, decreases stress, and boosts general well being.

4. Healthy Diet:

Adopting a heart healthy diet is essential for patients with CAD. Key nutritional guidelines include:

Low Fat, Low salt Diet: Reducing saturated and trans fats, as well as decreasing salt intake, helps regulate cholesterol levels and blood pressure.

Emphasis on Fruits and Vegetables: A diet rich in fruits, vegetables, whole grains, and fiber helps heart health by supplying critical nutrients and antioxidants.

Lean Proteins: Choosing lean protein sources, such as poultry, fish, lentils, and nuts, adds to a healthy diet.

Working with a certified dietitian or nutritionist can assist in the development of tailored dietary regimens. Making modest modifications and developing sustainable eating habits are crucial to long-term success.

Living with Coronary Artery Disease demands a complex strategy that incorporates lifestyle adjustments and medication management. Embracing a heart-healthy lifestyle, stopping smoking, controlling cardiovascular risk factors, engaging in regular exercise, and sticking to prescribed medications contribute to a complete strategy for treating CAD and boosting overall well-being. Regular follow-ups with healthcare experts, continued education, and a proactive attitude toward heart health are critical parts of successful management. The following part will address the probable consequences of CAD and options for prevention.

Complications and Lifetime Implications of CAD

Living with Coronary Artery Disease (CAD) entails identifying and treating consequences that might occur from this cardiovascular ailment. From the immediate long-term angina and heart attacks to the long term repercussions on the overall quality of life, overcoming CAD demands proactive measures and a complete approach to health.

Potential Complications

1. Angina:

Angina, or chest discomfort, is a frequent consequence of CAD. It happens when the cardiac muscle does not receive enough oxygen-rich blood, commonly during physical exercise or times of stress. While angina itself is not a heart attack, it serves as a warning indication that the blood supply to the heart is disturbed.

Addressing angina entails controlling underlying CAD through lifestyle modifications, medicines, and, in certain situations, procedures such as angioplasty or coronary artery bypass surgery. Regular contact with healthcare experts is vital for changing treatment approaches based on the frequency and severity of angina events.

2. Heart Attack:

A heart attack, or myocardial infarction, is a serious complication of CAD. It happens when a coronary artery is fully blocked, causing the death of part of the heart muscle owing to a lack of blood supply. The traditional indicators of a heart attack are crushing chest pain, shortness of breath, and perspiration.

Immediate medical assistance is important during a heart attack. Emergency therapies, such as clot-dissolving medicines or angioplasty, try to restore blood flow to the damaged region. Following a heart attack, patients may require continuing cardiac rehabilitation, medicines, and lifestyle adjustments to prevent additional issues.

3. Heart Failure:
Heart failure is a long-term consequence that can arise from untreated

or poorly managed CAD. It happens when the heart gets weaker and is unable to pump blood properly to satisfy the body's demands. Symptoms of heart failure include weariness, shortness of breath, and fluid retention.

Managing heart failure needs a mix of drugs, lifestyle adjustments, and regular monitoring by healthcare specialists. Individuals with heart failure may need to control salt consumption, maintain fluid balance, and participate in cardiac rehabilitation to enhance heart function.

Impact on Overall Quality of Life

The ramifications of CAD extend beyond the acute problems, influencing the entire quality of life for persons living with this ailment. Several variables contribute to the influence on quality of life:

1. Physical Limitations:

CAD and its consequences might result in physical limits, especially if there has been damage to the heart muscle. Individuals may suffer lower exercise tolerance, resulting in lifestyle alterations and adaptations in everyday activities.

2. Emotional Well-Being:

The psychological impact of CAD is important. The knowledge of living with a chronic disease, the worry of future problems, and the lifestyle modifications necessary can lead to stress, anxiety, and depression. Emotional support, therapy, and involvement in support groups are critical components of comprehensive CAD treatment.

3. Social Impact:

CAD can impact social interactions and relationships. Lifestyle changes, food limitations, and the requirement for medicines may need modifications in social contexts. Support from family and friends is vital for sustaining a pleasant social environment.

4. Financial Considerations:

The financial repercussions of CAD can be enormous. The expenditures involved with drugs, medical appointments, and other treatments might create a burden on financial resources. Individuals need to examine available resources, insurance coverage, and financial help programs.

5. Long Term Planning:

CAD demands long-term planning for healthcare and lifestyle management. Individuals are encouraged to engage closely with healthcare professionals to build tailored treatment plans that address their unique needs and risk factors. Regular follow-ups, preventative actions, and continual education are critical components of long-term planning.

The difficulties and lifetime consequences of Coronary Artery Disease underline the significance of a thorough and proactive approach to therapy. Beyond medical therapies, addressing the emotional and social components of living with CAD is critical for boosting overall quality of life. Empowerment via knowledge, support from healthcare practitioners, and a dedication to heart-healthy activities can dramatically affect the course of CAD and contribute to a satisfying and meaningful life. The third part will cover preventative methods, highlighting the importance of a heart healthy lifestyle in decreasing the risk of CAD and its consequences.

Emotional and Mental Health in the CAD

Living with Coronary Artery Disease (CAD) is not simply a physical journey; it deeply affects emotional and mental well-being. Recognizing and managing the emotional components of CAD is crucial to holistic care. In this part, we will cover ways for coping with the emotional issues connected with CAD and the necessity of support systems and resources.

Coping with the Emotional Aspects of CAD

1. Understanding Emotional Challenges:

A diagnosis can trigger several feelings, including worry, anxiety, irritation, and even sadness. Individuals may deal with the uncertainty of living with a chronic ailment, the dread of consequences, and the necessary lifestyle modifications. Acknowledging these feelings is the first step in effective coping.

2. Open Communication:

Encouraging open communication with healthcare providers is crucial. Patients should feel comfortable sharing their concerns, anxieties, and emotional challenges. Healthcare experts may provide assistance, remove misunderstandings, and offer comfort concerning the management and prognosis of CAD.

3. Educational Support:

Knowledge is a valuable tool for emotional coping. Understanding the condition, treatment alternatives, and the necessity of lifestyle alterations allows patients to actively engage in their care. Educational resources, counseling sessions, and involvement in cardiac rehabilitation programs can add to a sense of control and understanding.

4. Stress Management Techniques:

Chronic stress can aggravate CAD symptoms and severely damage overall health. Learning and practicing stress management practices, such as deep breathing exercises, mindfulness, and relaxation techniques, can be useful in decreasing emotional discomfort. These strategies not only improve mental well-being but also have good impacts on cardiovascular health.

5. Professional Counseling:

Seeking the help of a mental health expert, such as a counselor or psychologist, can provide a safe environment to explore and resolve emotional difficulties. Counseling can aid individuals in building coping mechanisms, controlling anxiety or despair, and creating resilience in the face of CAD related stresses.

6. Peer Support:

Connecting with individuals who share similar experiences may be important. Peer support groups provide a venue for persons with CAD to share ideas, discuss coping skills, and give emotional support. Hearing others' tales and triumphs may develop a sense of community and lessen feelings of loneliness.

Support Systems and Resources

1. Family and Friends:

Building a solid support network with family and friends is vital. Loved ones can give emotional support, aid with practical problems, and engage in lifestyle adjustments. Open communication within the family fosters understanding and joint decision-making around CAD management.

2. Healthcare Team Collaboration:

Collaborating with the healthcare team is vital for complete care. This team may comprise cardiologists, nurses, nutritionists, and mental health practitioners. Regular check-ins and updates ensure that the care plan matches with the individual's physical and emotional requirements.

3. Community Resources:

Many towns offer services for persons with CAD, including educational sessions, support groups, and wellness initiatives. Local health organizations and community centers can give information about relevant resources and events.

4. Online Support Communities:

The internet era has encouraged the formation of online communities where persons with CAD may connect, exchange experiences, and give support. Participating in these groups gives a virtual area for debates, information sharing, and mutual encouragement.

5. Patient Advocacy Organizations:

Patient advocacy organizations focused on heart health often provide helpful resources and assistance. These groups may offer educational resources, access to specialists, and activities that increase awareness and community participation.

6. Self-Care Practices:

Encouraging self-care habits is crucial for emotional and mental well-being. Engaging in activities that offer joy, relaxation, and contentment helps to a happy outlook. Whether it's hobbies, nature walks, or mindfulness exercises, adding self-care into everyday life helps alleviate stress and promote overall emotional wellness.

Addressing the emotional and mental components of living with CAD is crucial to a holistic approach to wellness. Coping techniques, support structures, and access to resources lead to resilience and better well-being. By maintaining a healthy emotional environment, persons with CAD may negotiate the obstacles of well-being with more strength and flexibility. The third part will cover preventative methods, highlighting the importance of a healthy lifestyle in decreasing the risk of CAD and its consequences.

Prevention Strategies for CAD

Prevention is a cornerstone in the therapy of Coronary Artery Disease (CAD), stressing the need for proactive actions to lower risk factors and preserve heart health. In this part, we will cover the relevance of prevention, practical measures to lower risk factors, and the value of frequent checkups and monitoring in preventing the beginning and progression of CAD.

Importance of Prevention

1. Proactive Approach:

Prevention of CAD entails adopting a proactive attitude to heart health. Rather than waiting for symptoms to appear, individuals are encouraged to adopt lifestyle choices and engage in actions that enhance cardiovascular well-being. Prevention not only decreases the chance of developing CAD but also lessens the possibility of consequences such as heart attacks and heart failure.

2. Lifestyle Impact:

The majority of cases are connected to modifiable lifestyle variables. Choices linked to food, physical exercise, smoking, and stress management have significant roles in determining cardiovascular health. By addressing these characteristics, people can greatly improve their overall risk profile for CAD.

3. Long-Term Benefits:

Prevention is an investment in long-term health. Adopting heart-healthy habits early in life and sustaining them consistently can have dramatic implications on cardiovascular outcomes. The cumulative advantages include lower incidence of CAD, greater quality of life, and a decreased probability of complications.

How to Reduce Risk Factors

1. Healthy Diet:

Adopting a heart-healthy diet is crucial to minimizing risk factors for CAD. Key nutritional guidelines include:

Emphasis on Fruits and Vegetables: These contain critical vitamins, minerals, and antioxidants that support heart health.

Whole Grains: Choosing whole grains over processed grains adds to greater overall nutrition and fiber consumption.

Lean Proteins: Opting for lean protein sources, such as fish, poultry, lentils, and nuts, decreases saturated fat intake.

Limiting the consumption of processed foods, sugary beverages, and excessive salt is also vital for maintaining a heart healthy diet.

2. Regular Exercise:

Physical exercise is an effective preventative strategy for CAD. Regular exercise helps maintain a healthy weight, decreases blood pressure, and adds to total cardiovascular fitness. Aim for at least 150 minutes of moderate-intensity activity each week, such as brisk walking, swimming, or cycling.

Incorporating both aerobic activities and weight training into the regimen boosts the total cardiovascular advantages. It's crucial to find activities that coincide with individual fitness levels and interests to achieve long-term adherence.

3. Smoking Cessation:

Smoking is a key risk factor for CAD, and stopping smoking is one of the most powerful preventative interventions. The advantages of smoking cessation extend beyond heart health and include improvements in lung function, lower cancer risk, and better general well-being.

Smoking cessation programs, nicotine replacement medications, and assistance from healthcare experts can aid patients in overcoming nicotine addiction. The sooner individuals quit smoking, the better the health advantages.

4. Maintain a Healthy Weight:

Maintaining a healthy weight is vital for heart health. Excess body weight, especially around the waist, is related with an increased risk of CAD. Adopting a balanced diet and engaging in regular physical activity contribute to weight management.

Healthcare experts can give help on setting realistic weight goals and making lasting lifestyle changes. Individualized approaches, focused on overall health rather than rigorous adherence to arbitrary body ideals, are crucial to successful weight control.

5. Stress Management:

Chronic stress can contribute to the development and progression of CAD. Implementing stress management practices, such as mindfulness, deep breathing exercises, and hobbies that promote relaxation, can decrease the influence of stress on cardiovascular health.

Engaging in activities that offer joy and relaxation, maintaining work life balance, and seeking help when required are key components of stress management.

Regular Check-Ups and Monitoring

1. Routine Health Check-Ups:

Regular health check ups are vital for maintaining general health and detecting risk factors for CAD. During these check ups, healthcare experts measure blood pressure, cholesterol levels, and other important indications. Early diagnosis of heightened risk factors allows for prompt intervention and preventative actions.

2. Cardiac Screenings:

Individuals with a family history of heart disease or certain risk factors may benefit from extra cardiac testing. These exams may include electrocardiograms (ECGs), stress tests, and coronary calcium scans. These tests assist evaluate heart function, diagnose anomalies, and estimate overall cardiovascular risk.

3. Blood Pressure and Cholesterol Monitoring:

Monitoring blood pressure and cholesterol levels is critical for CAD prevention. Elevated blood pressure and high cholesterol are substantial risk factors, and regular monitoring helps healthcare practitioners to make early modifications to treatment strategies.

Individuals with CAD or at risk of developing CAD may be administered drugs to reduce blood pressure and cholesterol levels. Adherence to drug regimens and regular follow-ups with healthcare practitioners are critical components of continuing monitoring.

4. Diabetes Management:

For patients with diabetes, efficient control of blood sugar levels is crucial. Uncontrolled diabetes considerably raises the risk of CAD. Regular blood glucose testing, medication adherence, and lifestyle adjustments are critical parts of diabetes care.

5. Lifestyle Check Ins:

Periodic lifestyle check ins with healthcare professionals give opportunity to review and reassess heart healthy practices. These check ins may contain conversations about food, exercise routines, smoking cessation progress, and stress management measures. Collaborative goal setting and modifications to lifestyle goals lead to sustained preventative efforts.

Prevention measures for Coronary Artery Disease involve lifestyle changes, frequent monitoring, and proactive healthcare participation. Empowering individuals with the information and factors build the basis for a heart-healthy life. The last portion will provide a complete summary of essential issues and offer

encouragement for choosing a heart healthy
lifestyle.

Conclusion

In the journey through the complicated landscape of Coronary Artery Disease (CAD), understanding, prevention, and proactive management stand as pillars of a healthy existence. This conclusion serves as a reflection, summarizing significant ideas and giving encouragement for choosing a heart healthy lifestyle.

Recap of Key Points

1. Understanding Coronary Artery Disease (CAD):

- CAD is a common cardiac ailment characterized by restricted blood flow to the heart owing to cholesterol deposits and inflammation in the coronary arteries.

- Risk factors include age, heredity, smoking, high blood pressure, diabetes, obesity, and a sedentary lifestyle.
- Symptoms may include chest discomfort (angina), shortness of breath, exhaustion, and, in extreme cases, heart attack.

2. Prevention Strategies:

Importance of Prevention: Proactive actions are vital for minimizing the risk of CAD and its consequences.

Reducing Risk Factors:

- Adopting a heart healthy diet rich in fruits, vegetables, whole grains, and lean meats.

- Engaging in regular exercise, aiming for at least 150 minutes of moderate intensity activity each week.

- Quitting smoking to reduce a key CAD risk factor.

- Maintaining a healthy weight through balanced meals and frequent physical activity.

- Managing stress with relaxation techniques and activities that enhance well being.

Regular Check Ups and Monitoring: Routine health check ups, cardiac tests, and monitoring of blood pressure, cholesterol levels, and diabetes help to early detection and successful management.

3. Living with CAD:
- Lifestyle Changes: Embracing a heart healthy lifestyle means stopping smoking, treating high blood pressure, cholesterol, and diabetes, frequent exercise, and adopting a balanced diet.
- drugs: Adherence to prescribed drugs is vital, with a full awareness of potential adverse effects and advantages.

4. Complications and Lifetime Implications:
- Potential Complications: Angina, heart attack, heart failure, and abnormal heart rhythms can develop from CAD.

- Impact on Quality of Life: Physical restrictions, emotional well being, social interactions, financial considerations, and long term planning are elements impacting the overall quality of life.

5. Emotional and Mental Health:

- Coping Strategies: Open communication, educational support, stress management, professional therapy, and peer support are crucial for overcoming emotional difficulties.
- Support Systems: Family, friends, healthcare team collaboration, community resources, online support networks, and self care behaviors contribute to a solid support system.

Encouragement for a Heart Healthy Lifestyle

As we manage the complexity of heart health, the road is not one of limitations but rather a quest for energy, resilience, and well-being. Embracing a heart-healthy lifestyle is a gift to yourself—a commitment to nurture the very center of your being.

1. Empowerment Through Knowledge:

Understanding CAD helps you to make educated choices regarding your health. Knowledge becomes a compass, leading you through the landscape of prevention, management, and resilience.

2. Proactive Measures for a Vibrant Life:

Prevention is not a passive undertaking; it is an active commitment to a thriving life.

Every heart healthy choice, from the meals you consume to the steps you take, contributes to the resilience of your cardiovascular system.

3. Strength in Adversity:

Living with CAD or managing its risk factors demands strength, but strength is not a lack of vulnerability—it is the will to adapt and continue. The path may involve hurdles, but each struggle mastered is a step toward success.

4. Holistic Well Being:

Heart health extends beyond physical metrics; it involves emotional, mental, and social well-being. Embracing a comprehensive approach to well-being guarantees that your heart beats not only with vitality but with joy, purpose, and connection.

5. Community and Support:

You are not alone on this path. Communities of support, whether within your family, among friends, or in online forums, encourage shared experiences, and a collective strength that overcomes individual problems.

6. Every Positive Choice Matters:

Every positive choice you make for your heart matters. Whether it's a brisk walk, a heart-healthy dinner, a moment of mindfulness, or a genuine discussion, each choice contributes to the mosaic of your heart-healthy lifestyle.

The journey toward a heart-healthy lifestyle is not a destination but a constant expedition—one where each step is a tribute to your dedication to well-being. Let your heart beat not just as an organ of survival but as a symphony of energy, resilience, and joy. Embrace the gift of a heart-healthy life, for in doing so, you give yourself the abundance of enjoying life to the fullest.

www.ingramcontent.com/pod-product-compliance
Lightning Source LLC
Chambersburg PA
CBHW032032290526
45786CB00012B/2522